Walking Logbook Jo
52 Weeks of Insights to Inspire

This walki

It is a record from _____ 20_____ to _____ 20_____

Walking for Health and Fitness
A health, fitness, and wellness website with books
and programs dedicated to walking and all the physical,
emotional, mindful, and spiritual benefits that come from
it to achieve a healthy, balanced lifestyle!

Walk on,
Frank S. Ring

Download the bonus content & supplemental resources for Walking Logbook Journal at:

www.walkingforhealthandfitness.com/walking-logbook-resources

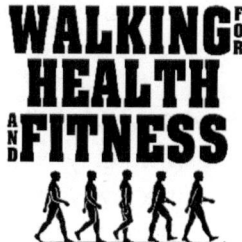

WALKING FOR HEALTH AND FITNESS

Contents

3   How to Use this Logbook – Journal – Idea Catcher
4   All Even Number Pages: Weekly Wisdom – Journal & Idea Catcher
5   All Odd Numbers Pages: Weekly Walking Log
108   Why Log and Journal Your Walking Experience?
110   How to Start a Walking Program – Develop a Routine
111   The 10-Minute Walking Time Test
112   Walking Safety Tips
113   Benefits of Walking
115   Things to Do While Walking
117   Develop Your Walking Creativity Routine
119   Why You Should Track These Vital Signs
120   Vital Sign Tracking Chart

About the Author

Frank S. Ring is a high school teacher and former track and cross-country coach with 21 years of coaching experience.

In 2016, he began walking to rehab from a back injury and fell in love with walking, to his great surprise. Frank has combined his love of walking with the website: **www.walkingforhealthandfitness.com** and has written three books about his passion:

- *Walking for Health and Fitness*, explains the benefits of the overall walking experience.
- *Fitness Walking and Bodyweight Exercises* highlight the benefits of bodyweight exercises
- *Walking Inspiration* is a 12-month plan to inspire your health and fitness with over 356 inspirational quotes and a monthly lesson to inspire your walking journey.

With, *Walking Logbook, Journal, and Idea Catcher* he helps readers capture the thoughts and ideas generated while they walk. Tracking your walking mileage is a motivator, and as you review your walking progress and reread your journal notes, you'll come to some fascinating insights on your health, fitness, and creative mindset.

Read more about Frank S. Ring:
www.walkingforhealthandfitness.com/about-frank-ring

How to Use this Logbook

A walking logbook shouldn't tell you what it wants to have in it; you decide what you want in it – what information you want to refer to and apply to future walks. I like this log format because if I choose only to walk, I have writing space to describe what I thought about, observed, and felt. If I decide to supplement my walking with bodyweight exercises or other fitness training, there's room for that too.

Distance, time, and location are typical of walking logs, but beyond those headings, you are the designer of this log/journal. You'll find plenty of space to record important information: how you felt, your ideas, your creative thoughts, weather conditions, what you wore, etc.

Each week you'll find insights to give you physical, emotional, creative, motivational, spiritual, and happiness pathways to explore. Walking has many benefits, and by walking, your world will open to many new experiences, places to explore, people to see, and adventures to undertake!

Use this logbook/journal to record your thoughts and others' words of wisdom to catch those great ideas that will emerge during your walks.

My favorite words of wisdom are from Brian Tracy, "Never consider the possibility of failure; as long as you persist, you will be successful."

I know you will persist in walking several times per week and utilize this logbook and its insights to their fullest.

I take your health and fitness seriously, and you'll see that through the words I have written and the care I have taken to put this logbook/journal/idea catcher together.

Before you get out and walk, please begin your walking journey by turning to page 108 and reading "Why Log and Journal Your Walking Experience."

Lastly, begin the biweekly tracking of your vital signs on page 119. Having a record of these numbers will help you quickly spot issues with your health.

Download your bonus content at:
www.walkingforhealthandfitness.com/walking-logbook-resources

This Week's Insight

What's Your Why?

Answer These Four Questions and Get to Your Why:

1. What happens if I don't walk?
2. What gives me "pep in my step"?
3. What are my strengths?
4. What fires up my passion?

Write down on paper or your Notes App the four questions then, go out for a walk. That's it; don't dwell on answering the questions, just let them be and see what happens.

Journal Notes – Idea Catcher:

MONTH			LOCATION	NOTES
	DISTANCE	**TIME**		Insights, Mood, Weather, Fitness Training
MONDAY				
TUESDAY				
WEDNESDAY				
THURSDAY				
FRIDAY				
SATURDAY				
SUNDAY				
Week		TOTAL	**Words of Wisdom:**	
Last Week's Y-T-D				
Year to Day		TOTAL		

This Week's Insight
Dramatically Improve Your Health in Three Steps

Step One: Drink more water - Your brain is approximately 73% water, so keeping your brain hydrated is essential. Being dehydrated by as little as 2 percent may impair your ability to perform tasks that involve motor skills. Drink at least 6 8oz. glasses of water daily.

Step Two: Get more sleep - Sleep helps your body repair its organ systems, including muscles, immune system, and other hormones. Sleep plays a crucial role in your memory system, enabling it to retain what you've learned throughout the day

Step Three: Breathe deeply - You trigger your body's natural relaxation response by abdominal breathing for 20-30 minutes daily. Inhale through your nose for about 4 seconds, feeling your abdomen expand. Hold your breath for 2 seconds. Exhale very slowly and steadily through your mouth for about 6 seconds. Aim for 5 x 5-minute sessions.

Journal Notes – Idea Catcher:

MONTH			LOCATION	NOTES Insights, Mood, Weather, Fitness Training
	DISTANCE	TIME		
MONDAY				
TUESDAY				
WEDNESDAY				
THURSDAY				
FRIDAY				
SATURDAY				
SUNDAY				

			Words of Wisdom:
Week		TOTAL	
Last Week's Y-T-D			
Year to Day		TOTAL	

This Week's Insight

It's Your Journey

Stop comparing yourself to others. Comparison places our focus on things and people outside of your control. It's your journey and no one can walk it for you.

Here are ways clear the clutter, end unrealistic comparisons, and make room for yourself.

- Be aware of your comparisons.
- Get to know yourself.
- Celebrate your progress.
- Speak kindly to yourself.
- Choose what you stand for and the kind of person you want to be.
- Be grateful for your efforts, lessons, and achievements.

Journal Notes – Idea Catcher

MONTH			LOCATION	NOTES
	DISTANCE	**TIME**		Insights, Mood, Weather, Fitness Training
MONDAY				
TUESDAY				
WEDNESDAY				
THURSDAY				
FRIDAY				
SATURDAY				
SUNDAY				

Week		**TOTAL**	**Words of Wisdom:**
Last Week's Y-T-D			
Year to Day		**TOTAL**	

This Week's Insight
Six Ways Inspirational Quotes Can Change Your Day for the Better

1. **Lessens the impact of a negative experience.** Reading inspirational quotes can put things in perspective.

2. **Gives you a needed lift**. My mom always used Robert Schuller's quote, "Tough times don't last, but tough people do." She said it so often that I thought she made it up! Let's face it, everyone will face tough times, whether physical, emotional, financial or whatever. For me, having this quote puts the breaks on my negative emotions spinning out of control.

3. **You're not alone**: Inspirational quotes remind us that the thoughts we have are a common experience felt throughout the ages. Your current emotion has been felt, discussed, and written about by others.

4. **Learning opportunities**: There is nothing we can't learn from. Seek out quotes on various topics.

5. **Keeps you grounded:** Inspirational quotes give a sense of the greater world around us. The thoughts and ideas of others give us wealth beyond money and bring us back to what is important.

6. **Gives perspective:** Picking up from the previous point, inspirational quotes help us get over the personal setbacks - from illness, loss, or a lack of confidence - we experience from time to time. By making it a habit of reading and writing down your favorite quotes, you can mitigate those downtimes.

Use the "Words of Wisdom" box and write in your favorite quote for the week

Journal Notes – Idea Catcher:

MONTH	DISTANCE	TIME	LOCATION	NOTES Insights, Mood, Weather, Fitness Training
MONDAY				
TUESDAY				
WEDNESDAY				
THURSDAY				
FRIDAY				
SATURDAY				
SUNDAY				

Week		TOTAL	**Words of Wisdom:**
Last Week's Y-T-D			
Year to Day		**TOTAL**	

This Week's Insight
Start a New Relationship with Yourself

See yourself as your best friends see you. Focus on your best qualities and fall in love with them. Remind yourself of your achievements, focus on the good you do for others, be kind, and believe in yourself.

On your walks, set aside a few minutes and focus on yourself. Image feeling deep and pure love for yourself. Picture a glowing orb of light sending warmth throughout your body. Bask in love and acceptance.

Journal Notes – Idea Catcher:

MONTH	DISTANCE	TIME	LOCATION	NOTES Insights, Mood, Weather, Fitness Training
MONDAY				
TUESDAY				
WEDNESDAY				
THURSDAY				
FRIDAY				
SATURDAY				
SUNDAY				
Week		TOTAL	**Words of Wisdom:**	
Last Week's Y-T-D				
Year to Day		TOTAL		

This Week's Insight

What Are Your Goals?

Answer these two important questions to take charge of your health and fitness.

- **What Are Your Health Goals?** Heal back pain? Lower blood pressure? Lose weight? Regulate blood sugar levels? Improve your outlook on life?
- **What Are Your Fitness Goals?** To be able to walk 30 minutes? To walk up the big hill in your neighborhood? Complete 20 pushups at a time?

Goal Setting Made Simple

These seven steps will get you to set your goals!

- Decide exactly what you want in terms of health and fitness.
- Write down your goals and make them measurable.
- Set a deadline.
- Identify all the obstacles that you will have to overcome to achieve your goal.
- Determine the additional knowledge and skills that you will require to achieve your goal.
- Determine those people whose help and cooperation you will require to achieve your goal.
- Make a list of all your answers to the above and organize them by sequence and priority.

Following these seven steps to accomplish any goal that you set for yourself.

Journal Notes – Idea Catcher:

MONTH			LOCATION	NOTES Insights, Mood, Weather, Fitness Training
	DISTANCE	TIME		
MONDAY				
TUESDAY				
WEDNESDAY				
THURSDAY				
FRIDAY				
SATURDAY				
SUNDAY				

Week		TOTAL	**Words of Wisdom:**
Last Week's Y-T-D			
Year to Day		**TOTAL**	

This Week's Insight

Ways to Stay Motivated

1. Create a Vision Board to help you visualize your intended results and allow you to see your ideal future. As you create the vision board, your creativity will begin to shine through and fire up your imagination as you literally create your future.
2. Break your goals down into smaller pieces.
3. Treat yourself whenever you have achieved these smaller pieces.
4. Share your walking goals with supportive people.
5. Keep yourself organized by having a walking routine.
6. Keep the big picture in mind.
7. Don't worry about what you can't control.
8. Seek out positive information.
9. Remind yourself why you set your goals
10. Be consistent!

Journal Notes – Idea Catcher:

MONTH			LOCATION	NOTES
	DISTANCE	TIME		Insights, Mood, Weather, Fitness Training
MONDAY				
TUESDAY				
WEDNESDAY				
THURSDAY				
FRIDAY				
SATURDAY				
SUNDAY				

Week		TOTAL
Last Week's Y-T-D		
Year to Day		TOTAL

Words of Wisdom:

This Week's Insight
Think STEPS to Increase your average walking speed.

Your capacity to move strongly reflects your health and vitality. **Shorter quicker strides**: Turnover rate is the key to quicker walking.

- **Toes propel you forward:** Push off of the toes of your back foot.
- **Engage your core and glutes:** Strong core muscles; the abdominal muscles, back muscles, and your butt muscles or gluteus maximus are essential to keeping your balance and walking well.
- **Posture:** Keep your body straight and your head up.
- **Swing your arms quickly:** An easy way to quicken your walking speed is to quicken the speed at which your arms swing back and forth.

Keep your focus on each of the 5 aspects of STEPS. Pick a point in the distance and consciously apply the STEPS in reaching the point. Eventually, as your body adjusts to the quicker pace, you will just naturally move faster.

Journal Notes – Idea Catcher:

MONTH	DISTANCE	TIME	LOCATION	NOTES Insights, Mood, Weather, Fitness Training
MONDAY				
TUESDAY				
WEDNESDAY				
THURSDAY				
FRIDAY				
SATURDAY				
SUNDAY				

Week		TOTAL	**Words of Wisdom:**
Last Week's Y-T-D			
Year to Day		**TOTAL**	

The Wisdom of Warming Up

The big mistake most athletes make is stretch their muscles before they are warmed up. Just like trying to start your car on a cold morning, your body must also warm up before you can get the most out of it.

The purpose of a warm-up is to

- Increase blood flow to your muscles
- Loosen muscles, joints, tendons, and ligaments
- Make you move more freely
- Cut risk of injury
- Get the brain engaged

The American College of Sports Medicine considers warming up an essential part of any type of workout.

Go to the Walking Logbook Resource page for a video of the perfect warmup:
www.walkingforhealthandfitness.com/walking-logbook-resources

Journal Notes – Idea Catcher:

MONTH			LOCATION	NOTES Insights, Mood, Weather, Fitness Training
	DISTANCE	TIME		
MONDAY				
TUESDAY				
WEDNESDAY				
THURSDAY				
FRIDAY				
SATURDAY				
SUNDAY				

Week		TOTAL	**Words of Wisdom:**
Last Week's Y-T-D			
Year to Day		**TOTAL**	

This Week's Insight

Add Interval Training

Research shows that interval training, workouts in which you alternate periods of high-intensity exercise with low-intensity recovery periods, increases your fitness and burns more calories over a short period of time than steady-state cardio, or in plain language, just doing the same thing for your whole workout.

For example, speed up your walking pace for a minute or two every five minutes. Or alternate one fast minute with two slower minutes.

An easy way to add interval training while walking is to pick a point up ahead such as a parked car or utility pole. Then, quicken your pace until you reach it. Slow down to recover, then pick another point in the distance and pick up the pace again. Repeat this several times during your walk.

Journal Notes – Idea Catcher:

MONTH			LOCATION	NOTES Insights, Mood, Weather, Fitness Training
	DISTANCE	TIME		
MONDAY				
TUESDAY				
WEDNESDAY				
THURSDAY				
FRIDAY				
SATURDAY				
SUNDAY				

Week		TOTAL	**Words of Wisdom:**
Last Week's Y-T-D			
Year to Day		TOTAL	

This Week's Insight
Odd Number Breathing Pattern While Walking

To breathe properly, you need to breathe deeply into your abdomen, not just your chest. Breathing exercises should be deep, slow, rhythmic, and in through the nose, not the mouth. The most important part of deep breathing is to control your breaths.

On your next walk, use my Odd Number Breathing Pattern:

- Begin by exhaling from your mouth for a count of 3.
- Then, inhale through the nose, thereby expanding the belly for a count of 4.
- The cycle is a 7 count (an odd number).
- Adjust the pattern as you see fit, but always use an odd number with the inhale 1 count more than the exhale.

Going forward, if you need to shorten the count-- especially if breathing gets heavier with more exertion-- just change to a 5 count: 2 counts exhale, 3 counts inhale.

Journal Notes – Idea Catcher:

MONTH			LOCATION	NOTES
	DISTANCE	**TIME**		Insights, Mood, Weather, Fitness Training
MONDAY				
TUESDAY				
WEDNESDAY				
THURSDAY				
FRIDAY				
SATURDAY				
SUNDAY				

Week		**TOTAL**	**Words of Wisdom:**
Last Week's Y-T-D			
Year to Day		**TOTAL**	

Step Up to Fitness Walking

What Exactly is Fitness Walking? Walking at a pace where talking to someone is labored. Fitness walking is the perfect low-impact way to get fit and stay fit! Because fitness walking is so low impact on your body, there is little risk of injury. When you are fitness walking, you can generally walk a mile between 14-16 minutes.

How to transition to fitness walking?

The following is an excellent way to transition to fitness walking.

- Within a pleasure walk, you pick up the pace for 5 minutes, slow down for 2 minutes, pick it up again for 5 minutes, slow down for 2, then pick it up again for 5 minutes.
- This will give you 15 minutes of fitness walking (approx. 1 mile)

How much should you do?

- Fitness walk 3-5 times per week
- Begin with 1 day per week of fitness walking
- One day will eventually become two days, two will become three, and so on, and so on.

Journal Notes – Idea Catcher:

MONTH			LOCATION	NOTES
	DISTANCE	TIME		Insights, Mood, Weather, Fitness Training
MONDAY				
TUESDAY				
WEDNESDAY				
THURSDAY				
FRIDAY				
SATURDAY				
SUNDAY				

Week		TOTAL	**Words of Wisdom:**
Last Week's Y-T-D			
Year to Day		TOTAL	

This Week's Insight

The Power of Your Brain

Exercise affects more than just your muscles. When you walk and do bodyweight exercises you are increasing your heart rate which pumps more oxygen to the brain.

- Exercise releases hormones that provide an excellent environment for the growth of brain cells.
- Exercise stimulates the growth of new connections between cells in many important cortical areas of the brain.
- Exercise has a positive effect on the brain's ability to change. This is commonly referred to as brain plasticity.
- Exercise increases the growth factors in the brain which makes it easier for the brain to grow new neuronal connections.
- Studies have shown walking 35 minutes on a treadmill increases cognitive flexibility which allows us to shift thinking and switch between topics.

The more you challenge your body, the more you focus your brain.

Journal Notes – Idea Catcher:

MONTH			LOCATION	NOTES
	DISTANCE	TIME		Insights, Mood, Weather, Fitness Training
MONDAY				
TUESDAY				
WEDNESDAY				
THURSDAY				
FRIDAY				
SATURDAY				
SUNDAY				
Week		TOTAL	**Words of Wisdom:**	
Last Week's Y-T-D				
Year to Day		**TOTAL**		

This Week's Insight

The Importance of Self-Care

Regularly hit the pause button and give your mind a chance to process all you've experience. Make it a daily priority to make time for yourself to sit quietly, breathe, and reconnect. Solitude gives us room to think, dream, nourish, and restore ourselves.

- Increase self-connection
- Reconfirm your goals and vision
- Build mental resilience
- Boost creativity
- Reduce stress
- Increase productivity
- Gain perspective

During this reset, breathe in through your nose for a count of four, feel your lungs inflate as your belly expands and chest rise. Hold for a two count, then exhale through your mouth for a count of six.

Journal Notes – Idea Catcher:

MONTH			LOCATION	NOTES
	DISTANCE	**TIME**		Insights, Mood, Weather, Fitness Training
MONDAY				
TUESDAY				
WEDNESDAY				
THURSDAY				
FRIDAY				
SATURDAY				
SUNDAY				
Week		**TOTAL**	**Words of Wisdom:**	
Last Week's Y-T-D				
Year to Day		**TOTAL**		

This Week's Insight

Keep a Gratitude Journal

Country singer Willie Nelson said, "When I started counting my blessings, my whole life turned around." End each day by writing down three things you are grateful for. You'll identify what matters to you and end your day on a positive note.

Use this logbook, gratitude app, writing journal, or create a folder of photos on your phone.

Journal Notes – Idea Catcher:

MONTH			LOCATION	NOTES
	DISTANCE	**TIME**		Insights, Mood, Weather, Fitness Training
MONDAY				
TUESDAY				
WEDNESDAY				
THURSDAY				
FRIDAY				
SATURDAY				
SUNDAY				

Week		**TOTAL**	**Words of Wisdom:**
Last Week's Y-T-D			
Year to Day		**TOTAL**	

This Week's Insight

Transform into a Problem Solver

Once you start walking, an amazing process of transformation begins to take place, you'll begin to think more clearly, you'll be calmer, and your creativity and problem-solving skills will kick into overdrive.

Try this out: As you prepare to go out and walk **(pre-walk),** think of a problem you are having. For example, I open my iPhone and create a new note on my Notes app. I dictate the problem at the top of the page then, I do nothing. I just walk, enjoy my surroundings, enjoy the feeling of motion, and enjoy the sense of accomplishing something.

Then, suddenly, my mind will drift over to that problem I put down on my Notes app. When I'm walking, I find my mind just randomly goes someplace other than where I am walking, and in this state, I begin to see solutions to problems I am having.

Journal Notes – Idea Catcher:

MONTH			LOCATION	NOTES Insights, Mood, Weather, Fitness Training
	DISTANCE	TIME		
MONDAY				
TUESDAY				
WEDNESDAY				
THURSDAY				
FRIDAY				
SATURDAY				
SUNDAY				

Week		**TOTAL**	**Words of Wisdom:**
Last Week's Y-T-D			
Year to Day		**TOTAL**	

This Week's Insight
How Leaders in All Fields Walk and Brainstorm
Walking to enhance the creative process is not a passing fade, great thinkers throughout history have used walking to facilitate their ideas.

- Aristotle – Walked the city streets with his students
- Beethoven – Walked with pen and paper in hand
- Sigmund Freud - Conducted many walking analyses
- Steve Jobs – Established walking meetings on first encounters with employees or business interests
- Charles Dickens – Walked up to 30 miles a day when working out problems with his writing
- Charles Darwin – Installed a gravel path on his property to walk and think through problems

If you are having difficulty communicating an idea to a colleague, head outside for a few laps around the local park. I have found this helps immensely in find creative solutions to our issues.

It is likely that the increased blood flow helps you to come up with more creative ideas and solutions to problems. Being out in nature and walking also helps you express those ideas more fluently and helps you to better communicate with co-workers.

Journal Notes – Idea Catcher:

MONTH			LOCATION	NOTES Insights, Mood, Weather, Fitness Training
	DISTANCE	TIME		
MONDAY				
TUESDAY				
WEDNESDAY				
THURSDAY				
FRIDAY				
SATURDAY				
SUNDAY				
Week		TOTAL	**Words of Wisdom:**	
Last Week's Y-T-D				
Year to Day		TOTAL		

This Week's Insight

Eureka Moments

A 2014 study from Stanford University has shown that people are much more creative when they walk around rather than sit still.

Set it and forget it

Eureka moments tend to come to us not when we're intensely focused on a problem but when we're idly thinking about something else, allowing our subconscious mind to chew on the issue in the background.

Because we don't have to devote much conscious effort to the act of walking, our attention is free to wander--to overlay the world before us with a parade of images from the mind's theater. This is precisely the kind of mental state that studies have linked to innovative ideas and strokes of insight.

Journal Notes – Idea Catcher:

MONTH			LOCATION	NOTES Insights, Mood, Weather, Fitness Training
	DISTANCE	TIME		
MONDAY				
TUESDAY				
WEDNESDAY				
THURSDAY				
FRIDAY				
SATURDAY				
SUNDAY				
Week		TOTAL	**Words of Wisdom:**	
Last Week's Y-T-D				
Year to Day		TOTAL		

This Week's Insight

Go with the Flow

Flow is the mental state of being sharply focused and engrossed in an enjoyable and motivated way. Do activities that help you reach this state, and you'll nourish your well-being. Often, we don't give ourselves enough time to do the want-to activities. We get so bogged down with the have-to stuff that we put our wellbeing off and never get to enjoy the pleasurable zone that flow allows us to reach.

- **Start small** – Commit just 10-minutes to an activity and focus solely on it. When you attention wanders, take a breath and bring it back to the activity.
- **Reduce the friction to doing the activity** – For example, if you want to write more, have a designated place with all your writing tools ready and waiting to be used. The quicker you can begin writing, the quicker you can reach find your flow.
- **Make time** – Get serious about prioritizing yourself and set aside time to pursue your soul nourishing activities.

Journal Notes – Idea Catcher:

MONTH	DISTANCE	TIME	LOCATION	NOTES Insights, Mood, Weather, Fitness Training
MONDAY				
TUESDAY				
WEDNESDAY				
THURSDAY				
FRIDAY				
SATURDAY				
SUNDAY				

Week		TOTAL	**Words of Wisdom:**
Last Week's Y-T-D			
Year to Day		**TOTAL**	

This Week's Insight
Walking and the Creative Process – Putting it All Together

In the pre-walk, you've written down the issues you'd like to explore or find solutions to a pressing problem. Now comes the easy part, walk and let go!

- Breathe: Start with the Odd-Number Breathing Pattern.
- Observe the beauty all around you.
- Create good karma for yourself by being the first one with a smile and wave when you see other walkers, runners, bikers, and passing cars.
- This is your time, use it to your best benefit.

Now the "magic" happens

It's usually later in the walk when the creativity I'm seeking begins to manifest. It may only be a fleeting thought, but when the spark happens, be prepared to capture it. I open my iPhone and dictate into my notes app all the ideas that come flooding into my mind.

The insight just happens, my mind will drift to the issue I'm seeking a solution too and it formulates in my mind; the next step forward; the missing piece of the problem; or the whole solution become crystal clear in my mind.

I'm still amazed at how often it happens that the ideas just pour out as I'm a block or two from home and often I'll say, "why didn't I think of this idea before", or "that was so simple, how did I miss it?"

Journal Notes – Idea Catcher:

MONTH			LOCATION	NOTES
	DISTANCE	TIME		Insights, Mood, Weather, Fitness Training
MONDAY				
TUESDAY				
WEDNESDAY				
THURSDAY				
FRIDAY				
SATURDAY				
SUNDAY				

Week		TOTAL	**Words of Wisdom:**
Last Week's Y-T-D			
Year to Day		TOTAL	

Improve Your Mind-Body Connection

Walking releases four vital neurotransmitters that impact your motivation, productivity, creativity, and wellbeing.

So why is this so important?

Neurotransmitters transmit electrical signals within the nervous system. Each of these neurotransmitters play a specific role in your emotional state.

- **Endorphins**: Natural pain and stress fighters.
- **Dopamine:** Motivates you to take action.
- **Serotonin**: Controls your mood and is responsible for happiness. It helps regulate when you sleep and wake, helps you think, maintains your mood, and controls your sexual desire.
- **Oxytocin:** The glue that binds together healthy relationships. Oxytocin release creates intimacy, trust and strengthens relationships. Often referred to as "the cuddle hormone," a simple way to keep oxytocin flowing is to hug someone.

One of the most exciting findings of the past few decades is that an increase in oxygen is always accompanied by an uptick in mental sharpness. Exercise acts directly on the molecular machinery of the brain itself. It increases neurons' creation, survival, and resistance to damage and stress.

Journal Notes – Idea Catcher:

MONTH			LOCATION	NOTES
	DISTANCE	TIME		Insights, Mood, Weather, Fitness Training
MONDAY				
TUESDAY				
WEDNESDAY				
THURSDAY				
FRIDAY				
SATURDAY				
SUNDAY				

Week		TOTAL	**Words of Wisdom:**
Last Week's Y-T-D			
Year to Day		**TOTAL**	

This Week's Insight
Staying Motivated Using a Logbook and Journal

Let's face it, life sometimes gets in the way of our hope, dreams, goals, and plans. Have you ever thought of giving up on your goals when the challenges you face seem too big to overcome? Our commitment to those goals and dreams are tested often. When roadblocks appear, it seems so easy to turn back.

How to Overcome the Roadblocks - Have a Goal

It's worth repeating from a previous insight that goals give us a purpose! If you have not set your goal yet, then set one now and get started on the road to successful walking! As Brian Tracy writes, "Goals allow you to control the direction of change in your favor."

Write It Down

Add as much information as you need to "paint" a complete picture of your walking health and fitness routine. I'm constantly added elements to my mileage logbook and adjusting my goals.

Fill in your information each day to monitor your progress. It's a great feeling when you look back 6-months from now and see, **in writing,** how far you've come as a walker.

The Journal will keep you honest. Having a blank entry will get you moving.

Journal Notes – Idea Catcher:

MONTH			LOCATION	NOTES
	DISTANCE	TIME		Insights, Mood, Weather, Fitness Training
MONDAY				
TUESDAY				
WEDNESDAY				
THURSDAY				
FRIDAY				
SATURDAY				
SUNDAY				

Week		TOTAL	**Words of Wisdom:**
Last Week's Y-T-D			
Year to Day		TOTAL	

This Week's Insight

Set a Self-Development Goal

Nurture yourself and you will grow. How do you picture your future? Do you consider how you would like to be as well as where? Would you like to be more confident and decisive? How about other character traits? With practice, these are qualities you can work on and develop.

Make a positive commitment to learn from and improve your life experience by setting self-development goals. Pick a goal, set a challenge for yourself and review your progress in a month.

Journal Notes – Idea Catcher:

MONTH			LOCATION	NOTES
	DISTANCE	**TIME**		Insights, Mood, Weather, Fitness Training
MONDAY				
TUESDAY				
WEDNESDAY				
THURSDAY				
FRIDAY				
SATURDAY				
SUNDAY				

Week		**TOTAL**	**Words of Wisdom:**
Last Week's Y-T-D			
Year to Day		**TOTAL**	

This Week's Insight

Celebrate Your Wins

You're a winner! But sometimes we get stress out by our day to day living which causes our confidence to wane, we judge ourselves harshly for feeling stressed, causing us to feel even lower.

Break out of this negative thought pattern by focusing your energy on your strengths and your achievements. Make a list of all the qualities you possess that you are proud of.

End your day by focusing on what you do right. Then, use the space below to make a list of your best qualities and read them often.

Journal Notes – Idea Catcher:

MONTH			LOCATION	NOTES
	DISTANCE	TIME		Insights, Mood, Weather, Fitness Training
MONDAY				
TUESDAY				
WEDNESDAY				
THURSDAY				
FRIDAY				
SATURDAY				
SUNDAY				

Week		**TOTAL**	**Words of Wisdom:**
Last Week's Y-T-D			
Year to Day		**TOTAL**	

This Week's Insight

Kindness

"Kindness is more important than wisdom, and the recognition of this is the beginning of wisdom." - Theodore Isaac Rubin, Psychiatrist

Kindness is a guaranteed way to feel good. Doing for others makes them feel good and is an action step for your happiness. Kind people feel happier. Increase your happiness and you're likely to be kinder too. It's a wonderful cycle as kindness and happiness complement each other.

Most importantly, be kind to yourself, you count! Be mindful of the way you speak to yourself, the time you give yourself to enjoy life, and your rest and recover. Being kind to yourself will increase your kindness to others. Keep your eyes open for opportunities for kindness, they are all around you.

Journal Notes – Idea Catcher:

MONTH			LOCATION	NOTES
	DISTANCE	TIME		Insights, Mood, Weather, Fitness Training
MONDAY				
TUESDAY				
WEDNESDAY				
THURSDAY				
FRIDAY				
SATURDAY				
SUNDAY				
Week		TOTAL	**Words of Wisdom:**	
Last Week's Y-T-D				
Year to Day		**TOTAL**		

This Week's Insight

What Brings You Happiness?

Happiness comes in many forms, such as laughter, joy, quiet reflection, memories, and anticipation of the future.

What does happiness mean to you? How do you experience it? With whom do you associate happiness?

Describe your happy place. It may be a real or imagined location, but imagine your happy place with as much detail as possible. Include sights, sounds, smells, touch and taste.

Whenever you feel stressed, take a deep breath and enter your happy place to bring your mind and body to a relaxed state.

Journal Notes – Idea Catcher:

MONTH			LOCATION	NOTES Insights, Mood, Weather, Fitness Training
	DISTANCE	**TIME**		
MONDAY				
TUESDAY				
WEDNESDAY				
THURSDAY				
FRIDAY				
SATURDAY				
SUNDAY				

Week		**TOTAL**	**Words of Wisdom:**
Last Week's Y-T-D			
Year to Day		**TOTAL**	

This Week's Insight

Exercise Your Senses to Stay Present

Bring your consciousness to the here and now by acknowledging your present experience through your five senses. Ask yourself the following questions:

- What do I see?
- What do I hear?
- What do I smell?
- What do I taste?
- What do I touch?

If you feel stuck in the past or future, do this several times daily until staying in the present moment becomes a habit.

Journal Notes – Idea Catcher:

MONTH			LOCATION	NOTES
	DISTANCE	TIME		Insights, Mood, Weather, Fitness Training
MONDAY				
TUESDAY				
WEDNESDAY				
THURSDAY				
FRIDAY				
SATURDAY				
SUNDAY				

Week		TOTAL	**Words of Wisdom:**
Last Week's Y-T-D			
Year to Day		**TOTAL**	

This Week's Insight

Understanding Stress

Stress is a natural reaction to the challenges of everyday life. In some cases, stress is beneficial as it pushes us to through life's tough situations such as passing an exam or meeting a deadline. But, serious stress on a regular basis can stop us from enjoying life.

Long-term Stress Symptoms:

- Aches and pains
- Insomnia and sleepiness
- Social behavior change
- Low energy
- Unfocused thinking
- Change in appetite
- Increased alcohol or drug use
- Change in emotional responses to others
- Emotional withdrawal

There are many things you can do to overcome stress. As you learned in a previous insight, walking helps your body releases four vital neurotransmitters. Exercise is a great way to trigger their release to relieve stress.

Journal Notes – Idea Catcher:

MONTH	DISTANCE	TIME	LOCATION	NOTES Insights, Mood, Weather, Fitness Training
MONDAY				
TUESDAY				
WEDNESDAY				
THURSDAY				
FRIDAY				
SATURDAY				
SUNDAY				

Week		TOTAL	**Words of Wisdom:**
Last Week's Y-T-D			
Year to Day		TOTAL	

This Week's Insight

Three a Day Stress Relief

It's important to make time daily to boost our mental wellbeing. Embrace the concept of doing three stress relief activities every day. You don't have to invest a lot of time or thought.

- **Get active:** Walking is a great stress reliever.
- **Eat a healthy diet:** Eat a variety of fruits and vegetables, and whole grains.
- **Avoid unhealthy habits**: don't deal with stress by drinking too much caffeine or alcohol, smoking, eating too much, or using illegal substances.
- **Meditate:** During meditation, you focus your attention and quiet the stream of jumbled thoughts that may be crowding your mind and causing stress.
- **Laugh more:** A good sense of humor can help you feel better, even if you have to force a fake laugh through your grumpiness.
- **Connect with others:** Instead, reach out to family and friends and make social connections. Overcome your instinct to isolate yourself.
- **Assert yourself:** Learning to say no or being willing to delegate can help you manage your to-do list and your stress.
- **Try yoga:** Through postures and controlled-breathing exercises, yoga is a popular stress reliever.
- **Get enough sleep:** Stress can cause you to have trouble falling asleep.
- **Keep a journal:** Writing down your thoughts and feelings can be a good release for otherwise pent-up emotions.

Journal Notes – Idea Catcher:

MONTH			LOCATION	NOTES
	DISTANCE	**TIME**		Insights, Mood, Weather, Fitness Training
MONDAY				
TUESDAY				
WEDNESDAY				
THURSDAY				
FRIDAY				
SATURDAY				
SUNDAY				
Week		**TOTAL**	**Words of Wisdom:**	
Last Week's Y-T-D				
Year to Day		**TOTAL**		

This Week's Insight

Slow Down

If you regularly find your stress levels are high, choose a daily activity to act as a break. Create a slow-down trigger that will stop you from your fast paced, get things done mentality.

Begin a ritual of taking a few minutes in the afternoon to make a cup of tea and slowly savor your drink as you take time to reflect on your day. Or, if you're at the office, deliberately clear your workspace. Slowly file papers, arrange your desktop items, and breathe deeply and calm your mind. Slowing down can have a big, healthy impact you your stress levels.

Journal Notes – Idea Catcher:

MONTH	DISTANCE	TIME	LOCATION	NOTES Insights, Mood, Weather, Fitness Training
MONDAY				
TUESDAY				
WEDNESDAY				
THURSDAY				
FRIDAY				
SATURDAY				
SUNDAY				

Week		TOTAL	**Words of Wisdom:**
Last Week's Y-T-D			
Year to Day		**TOTAL**	

Progressive Muscle Relaxation

PMR is the technique of tensing and then releasing each of the muscle groups in your body working from the lower extremities and ending with the face. By tensing the muscles, you can relax them more fully.

While inhaling, contract one muscle group (for example curl your toes) for 5 seconds to 10 seconds, then exhale and suddenly release the tension in that muscle group.

- Give yourself 10 seconds to 20 seconds to relax, and then move on to the next muscle group (for example calf muscles).
- While releasing the tension, try to focus on the changes you feel when the muscle group is relaxed. Imagine stress flowing out of your body.
- Gradually work your way up the body contracting and relaxing muscle groups.

With practice and time, you can learn to accurately identify stress and tension in your body.

Journal Notes – Idea Catcher:

MONTH			LOCATION	NOTES
	DISTANCE	TIME		Insights, Mood, Weather, Fitness Training
MONDAY				
TUESDAY				
WEDNESDAY				
THURSDAY				
FRIDAY				
SATURDAY				
SUNDAY				

Week		TOTAL	**Words of Wisdom:**
Last Week's Y-T-D			
Year to Day		TOTAL	

This Week's Insight
Walking and Affirmations

Developing a positive mindset is one of the most powerful and transformative habits you can include in your daily routine. Listening to affirmations while you are walking will multiply the effects of the affirmations.

Physical activity stresses our brain in the same way that it stresses our muscles. Like active muscle fibers, neurons of the brain break down then recover to become stronger and more resilient with exercise.

Affirmations are simply positive statements that describe a desired situation. "I am healthy, happy, and radiant!" is an example. It's a positive statement that describes your desire to be a healthy, happy, and radiant person.

Positive affirmations help your internal dialogue create a new vision of yourself and your life.

Affirmations are repeated several times so the subconscious mind can spring into action. Repetition is the key to reinforcing the learning and embedding the new thought into your mind.

Repeat the following affirmation several time a day this week: **I am talented with great creativity and intelligence.** Then have fun creating affirmations for yourself.

Journal Notes – Idea Catcher:

MONTH	DISTANCE	TIME	LOCATION	NOTES Insights, Mood, Weather, Fitness Training
MONDAY				
TUESDAY				
WEDNESDAY				
THURSDAY				
FRIDAY				
SATURDAY				
SUNDAY				

Week		**TOTAL**	**Words of Wisdom:**
Last Week's Y-T-D			
Year to Day		**TOTAL**	

Walking Meditation

Walking, combined with mindful breathing, is by far the most practical and easy to implement method of walking meditation. It has the added benefit of providing exercise for mind and body at the same time.

- Begin by moving slowly to find a rhythm to your movements and breathing.
- After you hit that sweet spot where movement and breath get into sync, you can move at any pace you want and walk as long as you like.
- Practice the 4-3 Breathing pattern.
- Inhale for 4 steps, exhale for 3 steps.

The goal is not to make it an effort, but to make it effortless and mindless... meaning that your mind is focused only on the activity itself and not the rest of your day, your problems, your work, or your to-do list.

The goal is to be fully present in the activity of rhythmic movement and breathing.

Journal Notes – Idea Catcher:

MONTH			LOCATION	NOTES Insights, Mood, Weather, Fitness Training
	DISTANCE	TIME		
MONDAY				
TUESDAY				
WEDNESDAY				
THURSDAY				
FRIDAY				
SATURDAY				
SUNDAY				

Week		TOTAL	**Words of Wisdom:**
Last Week's Y-T-D			
Year to Day		TOTAL	

This Week's Insight

Ease Anxiety with a 10-Minute Walk

Anxiety is a fear, unease, or worry that can be mild or severe. Our concerns grow out of proportion to a problem or situation. A sense of feeling overwhelmed can prevail, and we may not think clearly. Our thoughts may be irrational and even unfounded. Remember, negative thoughts are just thoughts and not necessarily based on reality.

Psychologists studying how exercise relieves anxiety suggest that a 10-minute walk may be just as good as a 45-minute workout. Some studies show that exercise can work quickly to elevate depressed mood in many people. Although the effects may be temporary, a brisk walk can give you several hours of relief.

Journal Notes – Idea Catcher:

MONTH			LOCATION	NOTES
	DISTANCE	**TIME**		Insights, Mood, Weather, Fitness Training
MONDAY				
TUESDAY				
WEDNESDAY				
THURSDAY				
FRIDAY				
SATURDAY				
SUNDAY				
Week		**TOTAL**	**Words of Wisdom:**	
Last Week's Y-T-D				
Year to Day		**TOTAL**		

This Week's Insight

Pet a Dog

Research has shown that simply petting a dog lowers the stress hormone cortisol. The social interaction between people and their dogs increases levels of the feel-good hormone oxytocin. Walking gives you plenty of opportunities to meet dog owners that are happy to allow you to pet their dogs. This is a win-win. You get to lower your stress level and maybe strike up a new friendship.

Journal Notes – Idea Catcher:

MONTH			LOCATION	NOTES Insights, Mood, Weather, Fitness Training
	DISTANCE	**TIME**		
MONDAY				
TUESDAY				
WEDNESDAY				
THURSDAY				
FRIDAY				
SATURDAY				
SUNDAY				

Week		TOTAL	**Words of Wisdom:**
Last Week's Y-T-D			
Year to Day		**TOTAL**	

This Week's Insight

Eat a Balanced Diet

Beat stress and fuel your next walk by consuming a good variety from across the different food groups, including fiber, protein, unsaturated fats and plenty of fruit and vegetables. Stress can affect our digestive system, but eating a balanced diet will help counteract its effects.

Journal Notes – Idea Catcher:

MONTH			LOCATION	NOTES
	DISTANCE	**TIME**		Insights, Mood, Weather, Fitness Training
MONDAY				
TUESDAY				
WEDNESDAY				
THURSDAY				
FRIDAY				
SATURDAY				
SUNDAY				

Week		**TOTAL**	**Words of Wisdom:**
Last Week's Y-T-D			
Year to Day		**TOTAL**	

This Week's Insight

Optimal Vitamin Levels

Keep your immune system healthy by including vitamins A, C and E in your diet. These antioxidants boost immunity and reduce inflammation.

- Vitamin A – Green leafy vegetables, fish oil, and eggs
- Vitamin C – Berries and citrus fruit
- Vitamin E – nuts, seeds avocados and olive oil

Vitamin B is another essential nutrient. B vitamins control production of tryptophan, which is used by the body to produce serotonin, the "happy hormone." Low levels of these can cause low mood and depression.

Boost your vitamin B levels with leafy green vegetables, broccoli, peas, chickpeas and fortified cereals.

Journal Notes – Idea Catcher:

MONTH	DISTANCE	TIME	LOCATION	NOTES Insights, Mood, Weather, Fitness Training
MONDAY				
TUESDAY				
WEDNESDAY				
THURSDAY				
FRIDAY				
SATURDAY				
SUNDAY				

Week		TOTAL	**Words of Wisdom:**
Last Week's Y-T-D			
Year to Day		**TOTAL**	

Break Up Your Busy Day

Busy day ahead? Schedule in some breaks and take advantage of them to help you reset for the rest of the day. Whether you set aside an hour for lunch or 10-minutes at a time throughout the day, think about what helps you recharge. It might be getting outside for a brisk walk, drawing, listening to music, or finding a quiet place to enjoying a cup of coffee. Give yourself conscious permission to relax.

Journal Notes – Idea Catcher:

MONTH			LOCATION	NOTES
	DISTANCE	**TIME**		Insights, Mood, Weather, Fitness Training
MONDAY				
TUESDAY				
WEDNESDAY				
THURSDAY				
FRIDAY				
SATURDAY				
SUNDAY				
Week		**TOTAL**		
Last Week's Y-T-D				
Year to Day		**TOTAL**		

Words of Wisdom:

3 Ways to Build a Strong Body and Heart

Add these three elements to you walking routine to supercharge your fitness.

- **Walk Faster:** Older adults capable of walking 2.25 miles per hour or faster consistently lived longer than others within their age group.
- **Walk Uphill:** Build balanced leg muscles, burn more calories, boost heart rate, and strengthen core muscles.
- **Add Bodyweight Fitness Exercises to Your Walking Routine:** By fitness exercises, I mean bodyweight exercises you can do while out walking. Your body will provide all the resistance you need for a fit, firm, and strong body.

Journal Notes – Idea Catcher:

MONTH			LOCATION	NOTES Insights, Mood, Weather, Fitness Training
	DISTANCE	**TIME**		
MONDAY				
TUESDAY				
WEDNESDAY				
THURSDAY				
FRIDAY				
SATURDAY				
SUNDAY				

Week		TOTAL	**Words of Wisdom:**
Last Week's Y-T-D			
Year to Day		TOTAL	

This Week's Insight

Walking and Back Care

Statistics reveal that over 80% of Americans will face some back problems. Lower back (lumbar muscles) strain and sprain are the most common cause of back pain. Your lower back supports the upper body's weight and involves moving, twisting, and bending.

- Back Health Benefits of Walking
- Strengthens the spine
- Conditions the muscles that keep the body in the upright position
- Facilitates strong circulation
- Pumps nutrients into soft tissues and draining toxins
- Improves flexibility and posture
- Nourishes the spinal structures
- Increases flexibility in your back and legs

Walk more and begin a back daily maintenance program.

Journal Notes – Idea Catcher:

MONTH			LOCATION	NOTES
	DISTANCE	**TIME**		Insights, Mood, Weather, Fitness Training
MONDAY				
TUESDAY				
WEDNESDAY				
THURSDAY				
FRIDAY				
SATURDAY				
SUNDAY				

Week		**TOTAL**
Last Week's Y-T-D		
Year to Day		**TOTAL**

Words of Wisdom:

Stretching

Stretching is an important part of any walking or general fitness routine, but please remember that stretching for 99% of the population is just to get to the point of moving freely and without discomfort. Stretching helps maintain flexibility, which is how far you can comfortably move your joints. Without stretching, your tendons shorten and tighten.

Flexibility is key to good walking posture. Good flexibility makes your moves more graceful, free, and fluid.

Walking for Health and Fitness Rules for Stretching:

- Hold each stretch for a slow count of 20-30.
- As you hold, take at least two deep breaths.
- Stretch **AFTER** your walk as your muscles will be pliable and more receptive to stretching.
- Focus on the muscle you are stretching and how it feels.
- Stretching should **NEVER** cause pain.
- Stretch to the point of mild tension.
- Pay special attention to muscles that feel tight.

Journal Notes – Idea Catcher:

MONTH	DISTANCE	TIME	LOCATION	NOTES Insights, Mood, Weather, Fitness Training
MONDAY				
TUESDAY				
WEDNESDAY				
THURSDAY				
FRIDAY				
SATURDAY				
SUNDAY				
Week		TOTAL		
Last Week's Y-T-D				
Year to Day		TOTAL		

Words of Wisdom:

This Week's Insight

Pick Positive People to Walk With

Walking with good friends or loved ones is a great way to de-stress. What could be better than laughing, feeling relaxed, and being yourself. The people we spend time with have a huge impact on our emotional well-being so pick positive walking partners.

Make your walking time your "positive energy" time. Share about the good that is happening in your life, include positive vibes, and ensure that the conversation goes both ways. Problems in life are unavoidable, and what better way to help you though them than discussing issues with those closest to you but. Avoid spending the whole walk going over your latest worries.

Planning things to look forward to with loved ones is a good mood-booster.

Journal Notes – Idea Catcher:

MONTH			LOCATION	NOTES
	DISTANCE	TIME		Insights, Mood, Weather, Fitness Training
MONDAY				
TUESDAY				
WEDNESDAY				
THURSDAY				
FRIDAY				
SATURDAY				
SUNDAY				
Week		TOTAL	**Words of Wisdom:**	
Last Week's Y-T-D				
Year to Day		TOTAL		

This Week's Insight

Try Something New

It's easy to get stuck in a rut and it can be hard to break away from our routines. However, making a change can be exiting and fun. Now is a great time to "think outside the box" to boost your mood and give a fresh perspective on life. Explore a new place to walk and find parks in the area that are tied to history. For example, I live near live near the Fort Lee Historic Park located on the Palisades cliffs overlooking the Hudson River, George Washington Bridge, and Manhattan. It's a great place to walk, and in the Visitor Center you can take a deeper dive into the Revolutionary history of the site.

Journal Notes – Idea Catcher:

MONTH			LOCATION	NOTES
	DISTANCE	**TIME**		Insights, Mood, Weather, Fitness Training
MONDAY				
TUESDAY				
WEDNESDAY				
THURSDAY				
FRIDAY				
SATURDAY				
SUNDAY				

Week		**TOTAL**	**Words of Wisdom:**
Last Week's Y-T-D			
Year to Day		**TOTAL**	

This Week's Insight

Make Hope a Habit

Hope is a feeling of expectation and desire for a certain thing to happen. Hope is fuel for motivation and a soother for anxiety and sadness. Making hope a habit is like a sensor light turning on when darkness comes. Hope acknowledges your strengths and capacity to cope when life gets difficult.

To cultivate the habit of hope:

- Get some perspective – Ask what the reality of my situation is, not my interpretation of it.
- Be persistent – Do everything you can do to cope with the situation. Including asking for help.
- Make progress – Take action! It may be difficult but without action you can't gain momentum.
- Have faith –Gives you somewhere to place your trust in times of uncertainty.

Journal Notes – Idea Catcher:

MONTH			LOCATION	NOTES
	DISTANCE	**TIME**		Insights, Mood, Weather, Fitness Training
MONDAY				
TUESDAY				
WEDNESDAY				
THURSDAY				
FRIDAY				
SATURDAY				
SUNDAY				

Week		TOTAL	**Words of Wisdom:**
Last Week's Y-T-D			
Year to Day		TOTAL	

This Week's Insight

Forgiveness is an Inside Job

Forgiveness gives you peacefulness and freedom. But, before you can forgive others for hurting you, forgiveness starts from within. If you can't forgive yourself, you will never truly understand the peace available to you. We've all got a laundry list of regrets that can keep us prisoners in our own head. Self-forgiveness is reminding yourself of your humanity, imperfections, and all.

Forgiveness frees us to be human, to be sorry, to offer apologies to others and ourselves, to correct mistakes, and move on with the intention of doing better next time.

- Forgive yourself for not wanting to forgive – Give yourself the time needed to be able to forgive.
- Practice letting go – You don't have to forget, but when you let go of what it caused, you bring focus back to your own healing.
- Make healing your priority – You have control over your healing. Focus on that rather than the need to get even.
- Forgiveness is a process – Allow forgiveness to be a process that take place over time. If you must, start with 1 minute a day to forgive someone.

Journal Notes – Idea Catcher:

MONTH			LOCATION	NOTES
	DISTANCE	**TIME**		Insights, Mood, Weather, Fitness Training
MONDAY				
TUESDAY				
WEDNESDAY				
THURSDAY				
FRIDAY				
SATURDAY				
SUNDAY				
Week		**TOTAL**	**Words of Wisdom:**	
Last Week's Y-T-D				
Year to Day		**TOTAL**		

This Week's Insight

Moving On

You can't change the past so don't let it spoil the present. You can learn from it and move on instead. Look at your what worries you and identify those that have roots in the past. Write these down on paper with a summary of what happened and how it made you feel. Read through your list and think of the lessons you can learn. Then, commit to bury them in the past and move forward with these new lessons and a positive outlook.

Journal Notes – Idea Catcher:

MONTH			LOCATION	NOTES
	DISTANCE	TIME		Insights, Mood, Weather, Fitness Training
MONDAY				
TUESDAY				
WEDNESDAY				
THURSDAY				
FRIDAY				
SATURDAY				
SUNDAY				

Week		**TOTAL**	**Words of Wisdom:**
Last Week's Y-T-D			
Year to Day		**TOTAL**	

This Week's Insight
Idea Catcher – A Bonus That's Free with Every Walk

Your walking time allows you to think. With all this thinking time, you will be amazed at the number of ideas that come to mind. Take advantage of this "bonus" and capture those great ideas before they slip away.

After your walk, while you are enjoying the endorphins still pumping through your brain, take out his journal and continue thinking, dreaming, and writing. I refer to this time as my "mind-dump" time. I like to write freehand. It allows me to mark up the page quickly with random thoughts that can be connected by drawing lines, shapes, etc.

It's essential to write longhand. There is a connection between the brain and the handwritten word that imprints the ideas and action steps on your subconscious mind. Typing out these post-walk thoughts is stifling. The red squiggly line of my typos is distracting. Pen on paper gives me a physical connection to my thoughts. It's a critical component that enhances the "mind-body connection."

I have the world's worst handwriting and I rarely write out anything longhand yet doing this exercise has me in love with this freehand writing process.

Journal Notes – Idea Catcher:

MONTH	DISTANCE	TIME	LOCATION	NOTES Insights, Mood, Weather, Fitness Training
MONDAY				
TUESDAY				
WEDNESDAY				
THURSDAY				
FRIDAY				
SATURDAY				
SUNDAY				

Week		TOTAL	**Words of Wisdom:**
Last Week's Y-T-D			
Year to Day		TOTAL	

This Week's Insight
Laughter is the Best Medicine

Laughter boosts your intake of oxygen, relaxes muscles, and releases mood improving endorphins. Laugher benefits your immune system and helps you get distance from your worries. Watch your favorite sitcom, go to a comedy club, watch comedians on YouTube, read joke books, or do whatever puts a smile on your face. If you're stressed, laughing may be the last thing you want to do, yet even a fake laugh will give you the same effects of real laughter and the benefits are just as powerful.

Journal Notes – Idea Catcher:

MONTH			LOCATION	NOTES
	DISTANCE	**TIME**		Insights, Mood, Weather, Fitness Training
MONDAY				
TUESDAY				
WEDNESDAY				
THURSDAY				
FRIDAY				
SATURDAY				
SUNDAY				

Week		**TOTAL**	**Words of Wisdom:**
Last Week's Y-T-D			
Year to Day		**TOTAL**	

This Week's Insight
Benefits of Listening to Audiobooks

- **You can listen while walking** - Audiobooks can provide entertainment, information, and help you pass the miles quickly. Nothing feels better than to end a good walk feeling physically and mentally refreshed.
- **Make doing tasks more pleasurable** - Doing dishes, folding laundry, watching your kid's little league game go into its third hour with no end in sight. Pass the time entertained with a good title. Who knows, you may hope for extra innings.
- **They're relaxing** - I Remember back to a time when my favorite teacher read a chapter a day at the end of class. I loved to listen to her soothing voice.
- **Faster reading pace = more books read** - You can set your player at 1.5 - 2x speed and it won't affect comprehension.
- **Helps you stay engaged with the book** - Exercise and learning go hand in hand. In fact, new research suggests that the real reason humans are primed to exercise is to support brain health! Studies have shown that aerobic exercise, can increase the size of the hippocampus.

Journal Notes – Idea Catcher:

MONTH			LOCATION	NOTES
	DISTANCE	TIME		Insights, Mood, Weather, Fitness Training
MONDAY				
TUESDAY				
WEDNESDAY				
THURSDAY				
FRIDAY				
SATURDAY				
SUNDAY				

			Words of Wisdom:
Week		TOTAL	
Last Week's Y-T-D			
Year to Day		TOTAL	

This Week's Insight

Quick Mood Boosters

If you're struggling to put a positive spin on your day, boost your mood with a quick fix:

- Commit a random act of kindness
- Dance and sing
- Compliment someone
- Be grateful
- Talk with a friend or loved one
- Add your mood boosters to the list

Journal Notes – Idea Catcher:

MONTH			LOCATION	NOTES
	DISTANCE	TIME		Insights, Mood, Weather, Fitness Training
MONDAY				
TUESDAY				
WEDNESDAY				
THURSDAY				
FRIDAY				
SATURDAY				
SUNDAY				
Week		TOTAL	**Words of Wisdom:**	
Last Week's Y-T-D				
Year to Day		TOTAL		

This Week's Insight
Intuition - Make Space for Your Inner Voice & Trust Your Gut

Intuition plays a major being in alignment with your core values and is key to living authentically. We may struggle with our intuition when we underestimate its power and when mistake in our past cause us to no longer trust it.

To harness its power, you need to make space where it can be heard and where you can accept it. On you next walk:

- **Get quiet** – Breathe deeply to quiet your mind. Try the Odd Number Breathing Pattern.
- **Let go of the external pressure** – Let go of the judgements, opinions, negativity, and press from others.
- **Listen** – Be patient and over time your intuitive voice will begin to emerge louder and clearer.

With any major decision, trust your first flash reaction. It's this "gut" reaction that shows your true feelings.

Journal Notes – Idea Catcher:

MONTH			LOCATION	NOTES
	DISTANCE	**TIME**		Insights, Mood, Weather, Fitness Training
MONDAY				
TUESDAY				
WEDNESDAY				
THURSDAY				
FRIDAY				
SATURDAY				
SUNDAY				

Week		**TOTAL**	**Words of Wisdom:**
Last Week's Y-T-D			
Year to Day		**TOTAL**	

This Week's Insight
Productivity – How Do You Eat an Elephant?

Multitasking sounds good in theory, but in practice it is fatal to productivity. Think how often you are doing four-things at once but none of them well.

Mindful productivity means training your awareness to be in the present moment working on the one most important task at hand. It means gently bring your attention back to that task when your mind begins to wander.

- Work on the one most important task.
- Work from a to-do list.
- Work according to your natural biorhythms.
- List the priorities in completing the task.
- Trust your intuition and take a break when needed.

Don't judge how much you get done each day. Taking small, consistent steps will go a long way to getting the job done.

How do you eat an elephant? One bite at a time!

Journal Notes – Idea Catcher:

MONTH			LOCATION	NOTES
	DISTANCE	TIME		Insights, Mood, Weather, Fitness Training
MONDAY				
TUESDAY				
WEDNESDAY				
THURSDAY				
FRIDAY				
SATURDAY				
SUNDAY				

Week		TOTAL	**Words of Wisdom:**
Last Week's Y-T-D			
Year to Day		**TOTAL**	

Why Log and Journal Your Walking Experience?

One of the best and least expensive wellness tools is a journal. Journaling helps you recognize and spotlight invaluable insights in your life.

Studies show that journaling is a powerful way to boost our mental health, reduce depression and anxiety, and make us happier and more content with our lives.

Benefits of Journaling
• **Reduce anxiety** - A 2018 National Library of Medicine study found that adults who completed a journaling session three days a week for 12 weeks were less likely to dwell on their anxious thoughts and better able to move past them.

• **Unwind and Sleep Better**- Spend 10 minutes focusing on your journal with all devices and screens turned off before bed. Anxiety causes sleeplessness, and by creating a to-do list, you'll reduce anxious feelings and drift off to sleep more easily.

• **Distance from negative thoughts** – Writing down your thoughts helps you consider them more objectively. Cognitive defusion is the idea that you are not your thoughts, emotions, or physical symptoms; instead, you are the context in which they occur. See yourself as separate from your thoughts.

• **Capture your creativity** – Capturing ideas and self-reflection are vital skills for creative types. It's also useful for entrepreneurs and busy executives, as it fosters clear thinking.

• **Heighten gratitude** – Gratitude raises our happiness, reduces anxiety and depression, improves physical health, helps us sleep better, strengthens our relationships, and makes us more resilient.

• **Stay organized** – Journaling help with decision-making, organizing your thoughts, focusing on your desires, and keeping track of tasks and obligations.

• **Clearing the mind through random jottings** – These brief informal notes and markings you write down help you make connections to a more significant point.

• **Track your mood** - If you experience an intense emotional response and don't know why then you won't be able to manage that reaction in the future. If you know what caused the episode, you can discuss this with your therapist and develop a plan to better cope.

• **Increase productivity** – Journaling encourages you to reflect on your work and work ethic and helps inspire new ideas to keep you on track.

• **Track the progress of your goals** – Life gets busy, and it's hard to stay on track. Using a journal can help you keep your goals in the forefront so you can accomplish them.

• **Improve memory** - By writing about your thoughts and feelings, you'll reduce the number of intrusive and avoidant thoughts throughout the day, freeing up mental space for memory.

• **One line a day to record one thought or memory** – Read these back at the end of the month.

• **Finding a Journaling Method** - Handwriting and typing work fine. Writing on your smartphone can work well, too. The critical issue is to put your thoughts and feelings into words.

If you need clarification on the advice on journaling, don't worry. The takeaway is that there is no right or wrong way to journal.

The best journaling practice is one that works best for you. Start with whatever method feels suitable for you. Start today; you'll efforts will be rewarded.

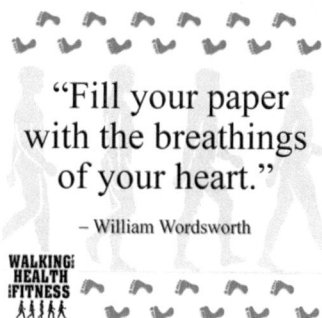

"Fill your paper
with the breathings
of your heart."

– William Wordsworth

WALKING
HEALTH
FITNESS

Download 20 Inspirational Walking Quotes:
www.walkingforhealthandfitness.com/walking-logbook-resources

How to Start a Walking Exercise Program

Starting a walking exercise program is as easy as putting one foot in front of the other. Start slowly and gradually work up to increasing the distance you walk.

As a beginner, aim for a certain amount of time, then set your watch and go. Enjoy the walking journey; it's well worth the effort.

The Warm-Up
The Biggest mistake most athletes make is stretching cold muscles. You will stretch after your walk. Doing a warm-up before you walk is easy and takes less than 5 minutes. I've included a video of my warm-up routine on the resource page of this book.

The Walk
You can walk almost anywhere! The important thing is that you walk.

Some suggestions on where you can walk:
• **Your neighborhood** - You know the terrain and the people. And by walking, you will get to know more people! I've met many new friends just by walking the same routes over the past few years.
• **A local park with a walking path** – Parks are quiet and not crowded with little traffic to worry about.
• **A School track** - An excellent option as you have a stable flat surface and can walk up the bleacher steps to get your heart rate up.

The Cooldown
Your muscles have been used and need to cool down slowly by following a routine similar to the warm-up.

Stretching
You will end by gently stretching your muscles. More details are available in my ***Walking for Health and Fitness*** book.

The 10-Minute Time Test

Walking speed is a powerful indicator of vitality: Walking speed studies shows that an older person's pace, along with their age and gender, can predict their life expectancy just as well as the complex battery of other health indicators, such as blood pressure, body mass index, chronic conditions, and smoking history.

IMPORTANT: The 10-minute time test:
- Choose a starting point.
- Begin your stopwatch (most smartphones have one) and walk at your normal pace for 10 minutes.
- Mark your endpoint to see how far you have walked.
- This is your baseline number, record it.
- Repeat this process every two weeks.
- Use the same starting point and see how far you can walk in 10 minutes.

By tracking your walking speed, you will be more aware of hidden health problems if you suddenly start to slow down your pace.

If you feel well yet have slowed down, there may be an underlying health issue.

The quicker you resolve the issue, the less time-consuming and expensive the treatment.

Keep track of your progress
Recording your walks in this journal is a great way to stay motivated and keep you moving forward.

In my classroom, I had fun using physical roadmaps to mark my progress as I recorded walking mileage in my walk around the perimeter of the United States.

Please read **"My Virtual Walk Around the United States"** on this book's resource webpage.

You now have excellent information on getting out the door and starting a walking program. Don't wait until tomorrow; start right now!

Walking Safety Tips

Please review the information in these videos to stay safe on the road this fall.

Walking Safely on the Road – Walk Facing Traffic
In this video, you will learn how to walk safely on the road by facing traffic These are the same tips I use each and every time to walk safely on the road.

Walking Safely with a Reflective Vest
Fall is upon us and the late afternoon walk could have you returning home in darkness. A reflective vest could save your life by allowing drives to see you more clearly. Think about how often you've driven at night only to see someone walking or crossing the road wearing dark clothing. They were nearly impossible to see until you were right upon then. Reflective vests are lightweight, can fit in your pocket, and are inexpensive.

Walk Facing Traffic
Knowing how to walk safely on the road will enhance your walking experience and keep you alive. Don't Become a Statistic – Walk Facing Traffic

For your safety, if you must walk on the side of the road, choose the side where you are facing oncoming traffic.

This gives you the best chance to see traffic approaching closest to you.

In Case of Emergency Medical ID
All smartphones have an In Case of Emergency Feature

Program your smartphone with your **ICE: In Case of Emergency contact information.** Also, fill in your Medical ID information.

In case of an emergency, your contact will be informed of your medical condition and precious time can be saved in getting you proper medical care.

We all think it won't happen to us, but an accident or sudden life-threatening illness can happen quickly. Better to be prepared and not to need it than to need it and not be prepared.

Benefits of Walking

Why am I so enthusiastic about walking? Well, I'll give you three reasons: it's free, it's easy to do, and it's easy on your body's muscles, joints, and bones!

And there's no question that walking is good for you. Walking is an aerobic exercise that stimulates and strengthens the heart and lungs, thereby improving the body's utilization of oxygen.

It also lowers the risk of blood clots as the calf acts as a venous pump, contracting and pumping blood from the feet and legs back to the heart, reducing the load on the heart.

- **Walking Fights Heart Disease** – With every step, walking is the best exercise for heart health. It can improve your cholesterol levels, blood pressure, and energy levels. Plus, it can fight weight gain to improve heart health overall.

- **Walking Helps Prevent Cancer** - A study led by American Cancer Society researchers has found that even low levels of walking were linked with lower mortality. Walking is the most common type of physical activity in the U.S. It has several biological effects on the body, some of which have been proposed to explain associations with specific cancers; including lowering the levels of hormones, such as insulin and estrogen; and specific growth factors associated with cancer development and progression.

- **Walking Helps Prevent Obesity** - Walking helps to prevent and decrease the harmful effects of obesity, particularly the development of insulin resistance (failure of the body's cells to respond to insulin) by reducing inflammation and improving immune system function.

- **Walking Helps Prevent Diabetes** - When you perform moderate exercise like walking three miles, your body taps into its stores of fatty acids for fuel more than it does when you exercise vigorously. That's good news for your diabetes risk, as an elevated level of free fatty acids can make it harder for your body to process the hormone insulin.

- **Walking Leads to Weight Loss** - A quick 30-minute walk burns 200 calories. Over time, calories burned can lead to pounds dropping.

- **Walking Helps Improve Back Pain** - Walking is a much lower impact activity than running. Most back pain is relieved with walking. By adopting a regular walking routine, you will strengthen your hips, legs, ankles, and feet, as well as your core. This provides better stability for your spine and helps to increase circulation in the spinal structures, draining toxins and pumping nutrients into the surrounding soft tissues.

- **Walking Helps Prevent Injury** - Walking improves range of motion and flexibility. Pain often restricts mobility. You will find that your posture improves as well as your mood. A stronger body and increased flexibility help to prevent injury. Walking at least three times a week for at least 30 minutes is great for overall wellness and a strong body. Combine it with a healthy diet and stress relief techniques, and you will look, feel, and move better – and your pain will be easier to manage.

- **Walking Improves Circulation** - Walking raises the heart rate, lowers blood pressure, and strengthens the heart. According to Harvard School of Public Health researchers in Boston, women who walked 30 minutes a day reduced their risk of stroke by 20 percent and 40 percent when they stepped up the pace.

- **Walking Stops the Loss of Bone Mass** - Walking can stop the loss of bone mass for those with osteoporosis. Recent research indicates that you must walk quickly to improve bone health and osteoporosis. Walking has been shown to improve bone density in the hip and femoral neck area.

- **Walking Lightens the Mood** - A California State University, Long Beach study showed that the more steps people took during the day, the better their moods were. Why? Walking releases natural pain-killing endorphins to the body which is one of the emotional benefits of exercise.

- **Walking Strengthens Muscles** - Walking tones your leg and abdominal muscles, even arm muscles, if you pump them as you walk. This increases your range of motion, shifting pressure and weight away from your joints and to your muscles, which are meant to handle the weight, helping to lessen arthritis pain.

- **Walking Improves Sleep** - A study from the Fred Hutchinson Cancer Research Center in Seattle found that women, ages 50 to 75, who took one-hour morning walks, were more likely to relieve insomnia compared to women who didn't walk.

Things to Do While Walking

I've come up with the top 29 things to do while walking. They've kept me walking, entertained, and in great shape!

1. **Workout** - You can create the ultimate fitness routine by combining walking and bodyweight fitness movements.
2. **Thinking / Brainstorming** - What's your most pressing problem? Walking has a soothing effect on the body and the mind.
3. **Day-Dream** - Getting "lost" in our own world helps you explore new ideas and helps aid your development and well-being!
4. **Pray** - Alone with your thoughts is a great time to get outside your head and pray.
5. **Walking Meditation** - My idea of walking meditation is to walk easily and breathe in an "odd number breathing pattern."
6. **Practice Gratitude** -Take a moment to acknowledge all you have silently. Giving thanks can transform your life.
7. **Learn Something** - Researchers have found that learning ability and memory retention improves because of the extra blood flow that walking brings.
8. **Listen to Audiobooks** - this is a fantastic way to enjoy a walk, pass the time quickly, and add to your knowledge base.
9. **Write Something** - You can voice your ideas into your smartphone. Start writing the great novel or that work email. Just download the text when you get home.
10. **Listen to Music** - Let the terrain of the road dictate your music.
11. **Photography** - You can easily carry a small camera or use your smartphone. Post your pictures on Instagram or Facebook while you walk!
12. **Track Your Mileage** - I've tracked my mileage for years and have walked enough to circumnavigate the United States.
13. **Scavenger Hunt** - Look out for particular objects. When I walk, I love finding coins on the road: how does a dime wind up in a small crack in the street?
14. **Reconnect with Family and Friends** - Use your smartphone by plugging in earbuds with mic capability; you can talk to anyone while you are out walking.
15. **Walk the Dog** (if you have one, or your neighbor's dog if you don't) - What better way to spend a half-hour than with man's best friend exploring the neighborhood?

16. **Enjoy the Environment** - Just being outdoors in the fresh air gives you a mental boost. Outdoor exercise boosts self-esteem.
17. **Walk with Friends and Loved Ones** - Does it get any better than spending quality time with the people you love and want to be with the most?
18. **Walk for Charity** - Many 5k road races allow walkers to line up at the back of the pack and walk the course.
19. **Have a Destination in Mind** - My long walks are to Starbucks or Dunkin Donuts. Coffee, snacks, and bathroom! I usually sit and write down my thoughts and ideas.
20. **Find your Happy Place** - It's that place that is yours alone, where you spend time with yourself. Mine is on a rock ledge overlooking the forest near my home.
21. **Walk in Pleasant and Enjoyable Places** - On the beach at the Jersey Shore is one of my favorite places to walk. Find routes that are both scenic and less congested.
22. **Discover, Explore, and Learn History** - I frequently walk in the Fort Lee Historic Park overlooking the Hudson River.
23. **Window Shopping/Mall Walking** - Walk a route that takes you through your town's main shopping streets.
24. **Do Yoga** - You can perform some basic yoga as you walk.
25. **Spread Happiness** - Over the years, I've noticed the more people I wave to, the more waves I get back. It wasn't long before people began waving to me first. I usually wave to any car that provides a wide pathway to walk. You can tell beforehand when drivers move to their left as they pass you. I always give these drivers a wave of thanks. I figure the good karma coming my way will help me during the times when fast drivers get too close for comfort.
26. **Rehearse a Presentation or Speech** - Do you have a big presentation or speech coming up? Rehearse it out-loud on the road during your next walk. Say it out loud with all the hand gestures you need to make a bold statement. No need to feel embarrassed; most people will think you are talking on your cell phone.
27. **Problem Solve** - I head out the door without thinking about the problem, then I just let my mind wander. I'm always amazed at how often the solutions appear, usually in the last 10 minutes of the walk.
28. **Community Service** - Clean up your walking route. Bring work gloves and a plastic trash bag with you on your next walk.
29. **Start a Business** – How can you start a business while walking? I've used walking time to brainstorm my books, website, and walking programs. My walking time allows for ideas to flow.

Develop Your Walking Creativity Routine

How would you like a boost to your creativity, mindset, and problem-solving ability and develop your Walking Creativity Routine?

"First comes thought; then organization of that thought, into ideas and plans; then transformation of those plans into reality. The beginning, as you will observe, is in your imagination." **-Napoleon Hill**

Walking and the Transformational Process
Once you start walking, an amazing process of transformation begins to take place:

- **The first transformation will be physical**. You'll begin to feel good! It will start slowly at first, then rather quickly; your body will begin to "feel good!" You will "feel" your body getting into physical condition. You won't be sore. You'll feel like your muscles have been used. Trust me; you'll want this feeling to continue. Soon, you will find that your average walking speed has increased as you become more fit.
- **The second transformation will be your mindset.** You'll begin to think more clearly. You'll be calmer, and your creativity and problem-solving skills will kick into overdrive.

"Yes, your transformation will be hard. Yes, you will feel frightened, messed up, and knocked down. Yes, you'll want to stop. Yes, it's the best work you'll ever do."- **Robin Sharma**

Develop Your Creativity Routine on Your Next Walk

- **Think of a problem you are having.** For example, I open my iPhone and create a new note on my Notes app. I dictate the situation at the top of the page then, and then I do nothing.
- **Walk and notice the surroundings**. Enjoy the feeling of motion, and the sense of accomplishing something.
- **Your mind will drift over to that problem when you least expect it.** When I'm walking, I find my mind just randomly goes someplace other than where I am walking, and in this state, I begin to see solutions to problems I am having.
- **Capture this insight when it hits.** Dictate into your smartphone or stop and write down your ideas on a notepad. Please don't leave it to memory. Ideas that emerge while walking are like dreams. Once you stop walking, they tend to disappear.

Stay Focused

Too often, we expend our energy on issues that have nothing to do with what we want in our lives. It's like being in a car race and constantly looking at the side mirror to see if the other car is catching up rather than focusing on what's happening in front of you.

A vision of what you want to achieve in life is necessary if you ever want to arrive somewhere. Stay focused on the goals you have set for yourself.

It starts by getting out the door

Athletes say the most challenging part of their workout is just getting out the door. When you create a "Get out the door" routine, you'll be one step closer (no pun intended) to maximizing your creative walking time.

- Ask yourself: "where will you be one year from now?" Do you have an answer?
- Are you still searching for your "why?"
- Are you on the right path?

"You're always one decision away from a totally different life."
- Anonymous

Your Next Step

Get out and begin walking today! I can't explain it other than when I'm out walking, I see the problem differently, and the creative ideas and solutions come quickly.

It's like a mystical process. I set the intention and let it go. Most times, the solution comes to me near the end of my walk.

Get inspired while you get in shape!

Why You Should Track These Vital Signs

Biweekly checking of your vital numbers can help establish what is normal for you.

You can share your numbers with your healthcare provider at your routine wellness visit. If you're not feeling well or notice changes, you can talk to your provider about them.

- **Blood Pressure** - Blood pressure monitors are easy to use, inexpensive, and available at grocery stores, pharmacies, and online retailers.

- **Weight** – You can use an at-home digital scale to monitor your weight, whether you're trying to lose, gain or maintain. Always weigh yourself on the same scale at the same time of day. Track your results so you'll recognize any abnormal weight loss or gain. Sudden, unintentional changes in your weight can be signs of an underlying health condition.

- **Pulse/Heart Rate** - Accurately recording your heart rate will give you a head start on detecting changes. You can relay measurements to your provider that seem different from what is normal for you.

- **Temperature** - Your temperature can rise if you are sick or taking medication that can trigger a rise. A home thermometer can provide important information quickly without visiting your health care provider.

- **Breathing Rate** - Sit calmly in a chair or on your bed, relax and count the number of breaths you take in a minute. A normal rate is between 16 and 20 breaths per minute for adults. Your rate is considered abnormal if it falls below 12 or rises above 25 breaths per minute. Abnormal rates can be a sign of a respiratory illness.

Tracking these five key vital signs at home can help you spot early signs of health Issues. If you notice any changes, you can talk to your healthcare provider and receive treatment sooner. An ounce of prevention is worth a pound of cure.

Download the Vital Signs Chart:
www.walkingforhealthandfitness.com/walking-logbook-resources

Vital Signs

Date	Weight	Pulse Resting Heart Rate	Breathing Rate	Temperature	Blood Pressure

Made in the USA
Thornton, CO
07/19/24 15:14:17

b14d40a2-5e6f-48d5-890a-0ba81f5665c9R01